20 lessons I learned in Dental Business Management

DR. GERMAN GOMEZ

D.D.S., M.D., Ph.D.

DEDICATION

To my beautiful daughter and wife, who inspire me every day to become a better person and a better professional. Their unconditional support is my biggest strength.

To my parents and brothers, whose constant faith, hope, help, and love have been a pillar for me through the peaks and valleys of my life's journey.

CONTENTS

CONTENTS

ACKNOWLEDGMENTS

I want to mention Dr. Bill Dorfman, who I met over 20 years ago, when I was a young dentist, and has been a mentor for me as a Cosmetic Dentist and as a person ever since. He has taught me a lot and still is there for me with valuable advice.

The contents of this work are intended to further general understanding, and discussion only and are not intended and should not be relied upon as recommending or promotinga specific method, diagnosis, or treatment by health science practitioners for any particular patient.The author makes no representations or warranties concerning the accuracy or completeness of the contents of this work and specifically disclaim all warranties, including without limitation any implied warranties of fitness for a particular purpose. In view of ongoing research, equipment modifications, changes in governmental regulations, and the constant flow of information relating to the use of medicines, equipment, and devices, the reader is urged to review and evaluate the information provided. Readers should consult with a specialist where appropriate. The fact that an organization or Website is referred to in this work as a citation and/or a potential source of further information does not mean that the author or the publisher endorses the information the organization or Website may provide or recommendations it may make. Further, readers should be aware that Internet Websites listed in this work may have changed or disappeared between when this work was written and when it is read. No warranty may be created or extended by any promotional statements for this work. The author shall not be liable for any damages arising therefrom.

Last but not least, when the author is writing about, and referring himself to the patient, the dentist or the dental team as "he", or is using the male version in an example, his intention is always to include the male, female and diverse genders.

1
INTRODUCTION

Dear reader, thank you for buying this book. The basic idea of this book is that dentists or physicians, who are like amateurs in the business field, get to have an entrepreneurial mindset. That means that in dental school or medical school, they have been prepared for their skills in dentistry and medicine, but not for business skills.

But as soon as they open up an office, they are automatically entrepreneurs. And at this moment, they need to have these skills. Either they learn them on the way and they make a lot of mistakes with that, or they buy books like this one.

The good news is, that in most of the countries, dentists compete against dentists that means amateurs compete against amateurs. But more in more and more countries, the system will be liberated.

And as soon as it is liberated, entrepreneurs are coming into the market. They will open up dental offices, chain offices, or similar companies. And this means that the dentist, that is established now, has to compete against real professionals (in the business field).

And although the system might not be liberated, it is not a bad idea to get skills in marketing, in sales, in closing, presentation and communication. Also in team management, and so on.

Because although you compete only against dentists or other physicians, it is not a bad idea to have an advantage in business. That makes you the leader. And this is why I wrote this book.

I am 25 years now in the dental business. Many years of them, in the beginning, I have been working in and with the dental industry. And when I opened up my dental office 16 years ago in Spain, which is a highly competitive market, because it is completely liberated 30 years ago, I had to find out the hard way, that it makes sense to own a set of business skills, and that you have a big advantage if you use this knowledge to make patients see and perceive, that you are a good option for them.

There are a lot of dental schools and a lot of dental chains in the market in Spain. And there I had to start from scratch. And I managed to make a really good dental office only by branding myself.

I would like to transmit information to all of you. Thank you again for reading this book, I hope you enjoy it and it opens your mind and provides you with some fundamental knowledge and ideas.

FUNDAMENTALS

2
HOW TO CALCULATE THE VALUE OF A NEW PATIENT

This lesson is about the real value of a patient. I mean a new patient. A patient, that has never heard about your office. This patient comes in because of your advertisement. How much is that patient worth?

The figures I will tell you are based on spanish prices and spanish numbers. You can make an analogism to your country using something like the Big Mac index.

The Big Mac index is used in the industries just to fix the prices in new countries where they don't know how to value their prices. That means I have something to sell like a dental chair, and I sell it in Spain for let's say 10,000 euros. Now I want to sell it in Nigeria. And I don't know how much I have to put the price on this chair.

So I will compare the Big Mac price in Spain and the Big Mac price in Nigeria. And then I can make an analogy. So that is what you can do for your country.

I give you a figure that you can compare with your country. The figure is for Spain: the usual price of a full ceramic crown is 380 Euros.

That is the price paid by the patient. The source is comparadentista.com, a platform to compare the prices of dentists in Spain. It is not my price. I don't say it is my price. It is the usual price in the market in Spain paid by the patient. It includes of course the materials, the sessions of work and the dental technician costs.

So based on this, if in your country, you charge for example, 760 Euros for you usually charge 760 Euros for a full ceramic crown, then you just double the numbers that I will write. Or if in your country the patient only pays 190 Euros for a full ceramic crown, then you just have to divide the numbers, that I will explain, by half.

So, what is the long term, the real value of a new patient?
What it is not: it is not what he pays in his first appointment. The patient comes through the advertisement, and it is not what he pays or spends on the first visit.
How can we calculate the real value of a new patient?
First of all, Usually, the patient will accept comprehensive care around 18 months after the first visit.
He knows you he got used to your clinic, to you, he trusts you, he trusts the way you are doing things. Now he is ready to accept comprehensive care. That's why we do not use usually the first appointment's amount of money that he spends. We start calculating the real long-term value of the patient.

Second: an average amount spent at the dentist per year, based on the years 2013 through 2016, is in Spain, around 500 Euros per year. The source: es.statista.com.
So, we know that in Spain, a patient as a mean value usually spends 500 Euros per year at the dentist. Some spent 6000 Euros that year, and the next year they only spend 100 Euros. But as a mean value 500 Euros per year are spent at the dentist, by every active patient.

That is a good number to know. Again, you make the Big Mac index analogy to your country please. I mean, if the patient pays 760 Euros (for example) in your country, then he is likely to spend around 1000 Euros as a mean value per year. And if the patient pays 190 Euros per full ceramic crown in your country, he is likely to spend as a mean value 250 Euros.

And we know also one more thing: the attrition rate of your patients. Patients who move out of town, patients who die, who change insurances, just change their dentist, and so on. This attrition rate is around 15% every year. Source: DentistryIQ.

We can then say that the patient is active in your clinic for around seven years, as a mean value. That is a very conservative assumption.

So, if a patient is seven years active in your clinic, and every year he spends 500 Euros, this sums up more or less 3500 Euros, that his value in your clinic.

That is why you should implement a loyalty system, just to make that these years become more, you can make out of seven years 20 years and then all of a sudden, his value is much higher. Then, if we do the math, seven years, active patient, 500 Euros a year would be 3500 Euros for that patient. But it doesn't stop there.

Because an average patient refers between two and five patients. That means if the patient himself has a value of 3500 Euros and he refers two new patients, that are also valued in 3500 Euros because they wouldn't come to you if it wasn't because of that new patient. So that value for both referred patients would be 7000 Euros.

And together with the value of this new patient (who became a referrer) it means business for you for 9500 Euros all 3 together (new patient and 2 referred patients).

But he if he refers five new patients, all of a sudden, all together would be 21,000 Euros. That is why you should implement a referral system in your office.

The resulting real value of a new patient, if he refers five new patients to you, during all these seven years that he is active in your clinic would be around 21,000 Euros.

Now you need to know, that if you spend 100 or 200 Euros in acquiring a new patient by advertisement, this one new patient might cost you 200 Euros but he will bring in business for an average of 21,000 euros.

You would be a fool if you would not do it over and over and over again.

3
DIFFERENCE BETWEEN MARKETING VS SALES AND FEATURES VS BENEFITS

What is marketing?

Well, in one sentence, marketing is everything you do, to bring a patient into your office, to make him call you, to make him contact you.

Marketing is everything you do to bring a patient in.
Advertisement,
offers,
your office design is also marketing,
the way you dress,
social media,
your website,
your logo,
business card stationery, that means your letterhead, a.s.o.
Your location is marketing,
front office protocols,
how they pick up the phone in your office,
how they answer the phone,
how they get the calls, and so on.
All the protocols in the front office.
Positioning of your advertisements,

also positioning of your clinic location,
your branding is marketing your message.
How you communicate your message out there.
Social proof is marketing.
Real reputation is marketing and so many things.

Sales is different.
Sales is everything you do face to face. If the patient is already in.

How is your office structured?
What's the first contact when the patient is in your office?
How is your front desk treating him?
How is your reception area?
How is the protocol of the first patient visit?
All these things are already sales.
How you inform the patient about the treatment options.
How you convince the patient to choose one or another treatment.
How you close the treatment, your closing techniques.
How you present the case to them.
Your communication skills, that shows your empathy.
How you listen to what the patient says and how you later take it into your case presentation or your communication. All this is sales.

When your marketing is good, the less sales you have to do. You have already sold by your good marketing, by the way, you get them in. For example, if you use social media, this is selling for you while it gets you patients in. If the marketing is very, very good, it's easy for you to open that shell later on during the sales process.

Feature versus benefit.

A feature is, what something does or has. For example, a crown rebuilds and covers a tooth.

Bleaching whitens teeth. That is a feature of the bleaching.

Periodontal treatment: the feature is, that it cleans up the pockets.

A crown is made out of ceramic Emax™, zircon, name it, that's a feature. Another feature would be, that it is a very hard crown.

Bleaching with a lamp or without a lamp.

Bleaching with 32% of hydrogen peroxide.

Periodontal treatment with laser, open or closed scaling and root planing.

The benefit is what it does for the patient. What does it do for him? What is the treatment of a crown doing for him? He can now chew without fear to break a tooth or something like that. Or he can smile without fear.

Bleaching: smiling the bright way. That's a benefit for the patient.

Periodontal treatment: no gum bleeding anymore, or no bad breath anymore. That's a benefit of the periodontal treatment.

What you want to do is in your marketing and sales message: you want to concentrate on the benefits, not on the features.

What's in it for him?

What does it do for the patient?

Create awareness of your patient's problem and then show how the benefit of your treatment can help.

4
WHY YOU SHOULD RAISE YOUR PRICES

This lesson is about why you should raise your prices and why this is a good idea for your office.

Competitive pricing is a bad idea. What does competitive pricing mean? Competitive pricing is to look at your market. How much is a crown for example? And you take the average price of it, and then make your price exactly like that average price. That's a very bad idea. Because who is then actually dictating your prices? Your competitors are dictating your prices, not you. They are deciding the pace of your growth. Not a good idea.

Competing on price is not a sustainable business model, there's always somebody else who can lower the price more than you do. And in the end, you don't have any margin, and you don't make any money. And you work the whole time.

Low margins mean more work, and longer working hours to achieve exactly the same thing as other dentists who have higher prices or bigger margins.

Business is based not on volume, it is based on margins.

Let me explain this to you a little bit more. If you, for example, want to make 1 million a year in your office and you are doing €100 treatments. For example, you're selling a crown very, very cheap: €100. Then you would need 10,000 patients per year to make 1 million Euros.

If you sell €1,000 treatments as a package, for example, then you only need 1000 patients that year to make 1 million Euros. But if you make packages of €10,000, then you only need 100 patients that year to achieve 1 million Euros.

On top of it to sell a €100 crown treatment versus a €10,000 treatment does not take 100 times more effort or 100 times more time to sell it. It is not even double the effort or double the time that you have to invest in case presentation and so on.

And if you raise your prices, you get more profits and less stress.

Second, to get 10,000 patients into your office to sell them a €100 crown costs a lot of marketing money and a lot of effort. On top of it, it takes a lot of your time to make 10,000 crowns a year.

---

1 Million / year

100 $ treatment – 10.000 patients – 1 M
1.000 $ treatment – 1.000 patients – 1 M
10.000 $ treatment – 100 patients – 1 M

Let me explain to you also why this is not a good idea to lower the prices, it's a much better idea to higher the prices. It is a matter of the margins.

If you sell one crown for €100, you need 10,000 patients to make the 1 million in volume. If for example, you take a very, very cheap dental technician who sells the crown to you for €60 then your margin per crown if you sell it for €100 would be €40.

You would gain gross €400,000 that year, only with the crowns gain, but with that you pay all your expenses except the dental technician, of course.

Now, if you make, for example, an anterior makeover with 4 crowns or 4 veneers. And you make them still cheap, for example, €250 each, instead of €100 each.

So, you raise the price more than double, but this is still not very expensive. You need only 1000 patients to do that treatment, as 4 times 250 equals 1000€ for the 4 crowns or veneers. You sell it as a package. That's the trick.

And now you can, for example, take a more expensive dental technician, better guarantee, better quality. Instead of 60€ you take a dental technician that charges 120€ and this dental technician uses better material, he is much better and it looks also better.

€120 times four for crowns or veneers equals 480€. Your margin in that treatment that you sell for €1,000 would be 520€. If you make it on these mentioned 1000 patients, you make 1 million of sales volume and your gross gain is 520,000.

So, you gross gain 520,000€ on 1000 patients, and before that, we calculated on 10,000 patients a gross gain of 400,000€.

Keep in mind, that you have the same expenses apart from the dental technician (who is already paid in this calculation).

Your gross gain is higher (and also your overall gain) and you work less although your crowns are of higher quality.

Example Crown

1 Crown - 100 $ treatment – 10.000 patients
- cost 60 – margin 40 – 400.000 of gain

4 crowns (anterior makeover) 1.000 $ treatment – 1.000 patients
- cost 120x4 = 480 – margin 520 – 520.000 gain

Upper smile makeover 12 crowns 10.000 $ treatment – 100 patients
- cost 200x12 = 2400 – margin 7600 – 760.000 of gain

Let's see another case, for example, upper smile-makeover 12 teeth and you sell that treatment for 10 thousand Euros, so you only need 100 patients that year to achieve 1 million.

Now you can select the dental technician. Take a good veneer or good crown for €200 each. You make the ceramic over 12 teeth, that's €2,400 that you pay to the dental technician.

So your margin on these 10,000 Euros is 7600. With one hundred patients your gross gain would be €760,000. Keeping the same overall costs, except dental technician (who is already paid in this calculation).

Do you see why that is a good idea at the end?

Now you only need to understand how to present the cases so that people see value in these €10,000. This is an issue of patient communication, presentation and sales skills. Watch out for other books written by me on these topics.

Also, the higher your prices, the bigger your margin. With this margin, you can now, of course, use better products to perform the treatment and to get better results. You can afford more marketing efforts to get these 100 patients in and a specific line of patients, a specific range of the society into your office.

You can add some extra value to your treatment, you have a lot of margin for that.

For example, spending some more time with a patient, or you can establish a VIP service or adding other low-cost treatments. For example, you can put into that €10,000 package a prophylaxis.

Or you add some more extra guarantee. Instead of 1 or 2 years guarantee, you extend to five years, six years, 10 years of guarantee.

Remember? You now use the best materials and technicians available and have more time to perform the treatment.

5
THE 4 MOST IMPORTANT SKILLS IN DENTISTRY

Few people in dentistry know how to communicate. Fewer people in dentistry know how to sell.

At the University they have explained to us the skills of dentistry to treat, diagnose, and to fix the problems of the patient's mouth. But usually, they don't teach how to sell and to communicate.

Nearly nobody in dentistry knows how to close but closing is the only thing that gets you money to the bank. You can be a very good presenter, and you can be a very good clinician, but without the close, you do nothing.

Skill number one is the ability to empathize with your patients. People don't care how much you know, until they know how much you care about them. You have to connect with the patient.

Skill number two is the ability to uncover challenges and discover your patient's pain points.

What does that mean? That means, if there is no pain for the patient, there is no sale. And this does not refer to physical pain, but much more like the "pain in the neck", i.e. psychological pain.

You need to make the patient aware of what he's lacking or what is concerning him most. He might not be very aware of that.

Don't sell, diagnose their needs, not their health status.

Of course, if there's something urgent to do with the health status, although they don't want that or don't really need that, they need to be treated on that, because it's your diagnosis that uncovers that issue.

But other than that, you need to diagnose the needs, you need to gather information about what they really need in their lives, about their problems and concerns.

Skill number three is the ability to handle objections.

The best would be to avoid the objections, but if you cannot avoid them, you usually start to be reactive to these objections. And if you cannot avoid them, you need to handle them.

Pre-discuss possible objections. You can make a list of objections, that the patients can make on certain treatments, implants, veneers, bleaching and so on, and discuss them, before he comes up with these objections.

But if other objections come up, then be prepared. Watch out for the Sales-Skills or Patient Communication Book, that I have written.

Skill number four is the ability to close. Closing is the only thing, that gets you money to the bank. If you don't close, you will do no dentistry.

No closing, no dentistry,
no closing, no treatment,
You need to close.

6
THE 4 DIFFERENT TYPES OF PATIENTS

Let´s talk a bit about the four different types of patients.

Everybody knows these types of patients, I just want to highlight them up a little bit, their features and show you what type of patients you want for your office at the end.

The first type of patient is called **"cheap" patients**. They are not really cheap, but you will understand why they are called cheap patients.

They are always asking about your price; how much do you charge? What is your best price? They are always bargaining. They are trying to lower your price.

They are always telling that they can get the same treatment somewhere else for less money. They don't really appreciate what you offer. They don't appreciate you. They don't appreciate your preparation, your education and your service at all.

What they want are cheap prices. They buy based on price.

The second type of patients is called **difficult patients**.

Difficult patients are not necessarily cheap. But what they have is a different attitude. They are negative persons, they have a bad day and they try to make your day even worse.

They ask a lot of illogical questions, it's not bad that the patients ask questions, but they should have a logic, they should be connected to the topic, to the treatment, but not questions, that challenge you in a bad way, in an offensive and tiresome way.

They are not pleasant people. They have negative energy. That's the difficult type of patients. They are very demanding. And it is really not worth the time you invest in the treatment that you do for these difficult patients.

The next type of patients is called **sophisticated patients**.

The sophisticated patients, have money, they are educated, they know what they are buying.

They have done research and they appreciate education. That means they are asking a lot of questions. But these questions are logic and they appreciate you to educate them.

The difficult patient already (thinks he) knows everything. In his mind, of course. Ask these difficult patients in what university they studied dentistry. And usually they say, I didn't study dentistry. Then you say, well, I have studied dentistry. Let me explain to you how this is going. They do not appreciate that, sophisticated patients appreciate that of course.

They need time to make a decision. So be patient with these patients, because at the end of the day, they appreciate that you invest the time to educate them and to explain to them the procedures, the alternatives, and the pros and contras.

And they also have a lot of questions but logical, intelligent questions.

The last type of patients is the **affluent patients**.

They have money, and they buy based on feelings. It should feel right. They don't need a deal. They don't ask: "Can you make me a 20% discount?", "Can you make me a two for one?". All these things. They don't need that.

What they want are other things. They want it to feel good. They want their decision to feel good.

You have to do everything you can to make them feel good

in your office, so that their decision, made in your office, feels good to them.

If it is cheap for them, something might be wrong with it.

They love exclusivity. One thing you have to have in mind is patients love exclusivity. If it is not for everyone, that's for me, I want it.

That is the type of the affluent patient.

You definitively want to sell and treat the type of patients, that is on the right side of this image. Sophisticated patients and affluent patients.

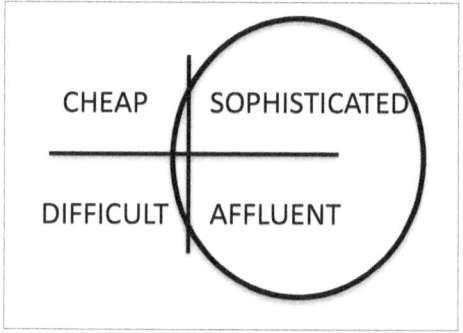

You do not want to treat and the left side, cheap and difficult patients.

How can you create more affluence of these patients? You treat them better. If you identify a patient, that is sophisticated or affluent, you treat him better. Better than the other patients, you stay more in touch with them. You send them more newsletters. Maybe you send usually twice or three times a year to all of them, then five or six times a year to the sophisticated and affluent patients.

You push referrals from their side, you ask them for referrals because an affluent and sophisticated patient might know other people who are all also like them.

You design your ads, you choose your language to attract them. You become comfortable with their needs. Try to subscribe to, for example, Robb report. Robb report is for very,

very affluent people. And they use certain language in their advertisements. They use a certain language in their articles and you get just very used to what an affluent and sophisticated patient has as interests. And you can cater to that later.

Don't make any discounts to the left side of the image (cheap and difficult patients).

If they want to be treated by you they will pay your price.

Do not make any discounts in general. But that is a whole other issue.

PERSONAL BRANDING

7
THE DIFFERENCE BETWEEN YOUR OFFICE MISSION AND VISION STATEMENT

We want to talk about the difference between your mission statement and your vision statement for your office.

The mission statement answers the questions why do we exist? Whereas the vision statement answers the question: Where are we going to?

Mission Statement

Why do we exist?

Vision Statement

Where are we going to?

First let me explain to you why it is important that you have a mission statement and a vision statement. It does pay off to have these statements. A Harvard study across 20 Industries found companies with vision statements had four times more revenue creation, seven times more job creation, 12 times faster stock price growth, and 750% higher profits.

Newsweek looked at 1000 companies and found those with vision statements had a 16.1% average return on stockholder equity, compared to those who did not have a statement, had only a 7.9% return on stockholder equity.

And, at last, but not least, those two last looked at €1 investment in 1926. Companies with a vision statement returned €6,350, companies without a vision statement return €950 only.

Mission Statement

What is a mission statement? A mission statement answers the question: why do we exist? Mission statements are foundational. The components of a mission statement are as follows.

We start with for example, "Our mission is", to then explain what we do, for whom we do it, so that we can describe our ideal patients and what is the benefit these patients or the world gets from our existence.

Let's make a checklist for a great mission statement.
It needs to be original, not copied.
It needs to be foundational.
It should sustain over time, you shouldn't change it every other month for example,
and your staff should know that their purpose and reason they come to work is expressed in the statement.
It needs to be original.
It needs to be memorable, short and concise.

It should fit on a T-shirt and your staff should be willing to wear it.

How to write a mission statement? Get ideas from your staff. They know you and the office well. With that input, create three or four versions and vote or pick one.

Here's an example I took from an ad from a Google search, which has more or less all these components. It reads:

"Our mission is to help our patients to accept the best care possible and to invest in dentistry, that provides their lives."

This example, from a google search, has more or less all these components.

It starts with "our mission". what is the mission? What do they do? They help their patients, and they help their patients to accept the best care possible.

And what's the benefit? Well, these patients invest in dentistry and their lives are improved.

They don't describe exactly who their patients are. Having stated that, now we talk about the vision statement.

Vision Statement

Where are we going to? It is about creating a different future. And this future is described in the vision statement. This future is different from how the situation is now.

Now we are at one point in our development, of our clinic, of our office, and in the future, we want it to be different. That's our vision.

There are different types of vision statements:

Quantitative:
They can be quantitative like numbers. Measurable like we want to do 2000 implants per year or we want to see 4000 new patients in three years or something like that.

Competitive:
It could be like beating the competition. Being better than a reference office or company.

I would definitely not suggest having a competitive vision statement, because it is kind of negative.

Superlative:
Superlative means we want to be the best, the number one, the premier, or similar.

Let's see, what are the components of a vision statement:

It starts with "We envision" you can take that statement away later. But start with that, then state your impact.

What is your impact? It describes what will be different through you, for your patients, for the world.

And then, what the world, your patient's life or what you described would be different, would look like after you have transformed it, or what your office would look like after you have transformed it.

And then include a year number like "in 10 years from now" or "by 2030" we will be like that, or it will be like that.

Vision statement checklist:
It should contain five or more years from now, so it should be written in a future tense.

It should be directional, we are not there today.

You have to think big.

It should be descriptive. Create a picture, how will it look like?

Here's another example I took from the internet from a Google search.

"The vision I have for XYZ-Dental is to have an office that provides the highest level of dental care to patients. We will help them make educated decisions about the treatment goals. Treatment will be painless, affordable, educational, among others. Ultimately, we will take the fear out of visiting the dentist. We will work as a team to make every dental visit the most comfortable, enjoyable experience possible."

It states "we envision", then what will be different. In this case it will be different because the treatments will be painless, affordable, educational and without fear.

They do not describe when they want to achieve this goal, but it is at least a vision statement for this office.

My last advice: focus on the future you cannot lead an office if you don't have a vision.

8
FUNDAMENTALS OF PERSONAL BRANDING FOR DENTISTS

I want to talk to you about the fundamentals of personal branding for dentists.

First of all, we have to talk about definitions.

Marketing is everything you do to bring a patient in or keep him or her.

Sales is everything you do face to face; your lips are moving.

Every time your lips are moving, and a patient is present, you are selling. You may be aware of it or not. But that's how it is. See also the chapter difference between marketing and sales for more information about this issue.

Branding is influencing the opinion of others about you. It is an enduring perception of you. You project your brand to others. It is the impression, that you have on others.

Ask yourself: Do you have a personal brand right now?

Of course, you have. Everybody is talking. People are talking about you. They are talking about you face to face, they are talking about you on the internet.

You need to guide these conversations into a direction that

you want them to. That means, how do you want them to perceive you?

Branding is influencing. It appeals to our desires and touches our emotions. It is more emotional. The goal is to emotionally predispose patients into entering a relationship with you.

At first, they don't know you. But the image that you reflect, appeals to them. The challenge is to ask yourself how you become more of people's dentist of choice before they even need one.

You would be their dentist of choice, but at that moment, they don't need on. But as soon as they need one, you would be the first, who comes into their mind. That's branding.

That's what it means to be in the mind or to have a positive image.

That personal image is not a personal brand. A personal image is what people instantly see. What they perceive at a glance, the way you dress, among other things.

The personal brand is what they think of you long term. That's your reputation. A personal brand is about creating a unique personal identity around a leading attribute, something you do very well. For example, you are a very nice or a very good smile designer. Then make your whole brand identity around that.

Managing the perception of your community. How they perceive you. You should try to make them feel a certain way about you. Your treatments: they should think, when you touch their teeth it would feel very good. It should be you who touches their teeth and not anybody else.

If it comes to smile design, if it comes to orthodontics, if it comes to their bleeding gums, you should be their choice.

A personal brand pre-sells potential patients on you, before they even meet you. They are already pre-sold when they come to your office. Then it is up to you to explain to them the options they have, and they do it with you.

Everything you do affects your personal brand:

- The way you walk, dress and talk,
- your education,
- your neighborhood,
- your specialties,
- the way you sell,
- the way you negotiate,
- your customer service,
- your presentation skills, and
- how well you follow through all your promises.

That builds your personal brand.

Where does a personal brand begin? You have to ask yourself:

- Am I perceived as I want to be perceived?
- What is my reputation in town?
- Does my brand reflect most my personality or my abilities right now?
- The logo you have, what's your personal brand right now?
- What makes me unique?

And just go and highlighten that a little bit.

- Does my website or social media channels reflect my brand?
- Are they on the same level? Are they on the same page?

How to systematically build a personal branding or brand authority? You have to ask yourself what you want to be known for. For example: I want to be known as the best, or as the cheapest, as the most expensive, as the most exclusive dentist in town. What do you want to be known for? That's your brand. That's your personal brand.

The last thing you want is, to appear as another dentist, just another one. No, you want to be special. You want to have a brand, then you are in the mind of the potential patients before they even need a dentist.

Start calling yourself an expert in, don't wait for permission, claim the position then back it up.

You need to own the website of your name or your specialty in your city.com. For example, smilevalencia.com or smiledesignerchicago.com. The ".com" is very important.

9
HOW TO WRITE YOUR
PERSONAL ELEVATOR PITCH

This chapter will talk about how to write your personal elevator pitch. And we will learn what it is and what it's not. You will learn steps to write an elevator pitch, I will show you a template and an example of how to write your elevator pitch, and I will point out the mistakes you have to avoid.

You meet someone at the restaurant, in a networking event, in the gym, and they ask: What do you do for a living? Whatever you do, don't just say "I'm a dentist".

The response you'll usually get range from "Oh, I hate dentists" to "Does this look infected?". You don't want that.

Instead, see this as an opportunity to promote your skills and generate interest in the business world. This is called having an elevator pitch.

What is an elevator pitch? It is a powerful representation of who you are. It is short, an engaging introduction to you, and the value you offer.

And it tells someone why they should want to choose you as a dentist. What's the purpose? It is to quickly let others know what your expertise is, and what your greatest accomplishments are.

- It is very short.
- It is between 20 and 60 seconds. Best thing is under 30 seconds.
- It is goal-oriented.
- It is personal.
- It is about you. (It's not really about you, you will understand me later.) It's about what you can offer to others.
- It is specific and targeted.
- And It should be interesting.

What it should not be:
- It should not be a review of your resume.
- It should not be a list of your skills and strengths.
- And it should not be a request for a patient to come to your office.

He will naturally know that you are the correct person, and he will naturally choose you. It is more about what you have to offer to the listener.

It is not that you are a dentist. You should not say just that. But what should you say?

Lots of things get attention but only two things get interest. You want to get the interest of the person that listens to you when you make that talk, when you give that elevator pitch.

First of all, people are interested if they have a problem that they don't want, and a result they want, that they don't have. Let me repeat that.

People are interested when it comes to talking about a problem they have, they don't want, and about a result they want and they don't have.

If you have that in your elevator pitch, they are focused and they listen to you.

It is all about outcomes. Potential patients don't care about the work you do. They don't care about who you are. They don't care about how great you are. They only care about the outcome you can help them create. That's what they care about.

So, focus on the most awesome, most powerful outcome that you provide as a pure dentist, as an orthodontist, as an esthetic dentist, as a general dentist, as a pedodontist, as a root canal specialist.

Build 100% of your messages, also the elevator pitch, around that. Advertisement, marketing, everything.

Step two, write your elevator pitch.

First, identify who you are, and who you help.

Second, identify your why. Why you do what you do. Write that down. Write down who you help, write down why you do what you do. Your purpose, your passion, your commitment. Why you're passionate about what you do.

You will take elements of what you wrote down to make your elevator pitch. You can start with "One of my greatest passions is".

Third, what makes you unique or special? Your greatest accomplishments, the largest problems you have solved. Major contributions you have made, how many patients you have already treated? What's your background? Something special, something that makes you unique.

And fourth, after all, include a call to action. No elevator pitch without a call to action, or question at the end.

And then practice, practice, practice, practice and revise and change. Don't be afraid to change it. Practice with family members, with friends, with colleagues.

Here is a template for your elevator pitch:

Hi, my name is X.

I'm an orthodontist, (dentist, periodontist, ...) helping (the people you help and the pains you solve).

I'm passionate about X

I've been fortunate to (your biggest problems that you have solved or the greatest accomplishment that make you special)

Have you ever (then a question or a call to action)?

Let me show you an example.

"Hi, my name is Peter Smith.

I'm a smile creating dentist helping people who are unhappy with the appearance of their teeth.

My greatest passion is to design and build the exclusive smiles of their dreams they love and enjoy.

I've been fortunate to have gone through years of aesthetic dentistry and dental implants training to be able to help over 5000 patients from all over the world to smile again.

Have you ever thought about enhancing your smile?

This pitch is under 30 seconds and it is about really having all the elements of an elevator pitch you can change it towards your personal experience, your personal situation.

And here is what you have to avoid:
-   Speaking too fast. Yes, you only have 60 seconds or 30 seconds, but try to avoid cramming 15 minutes in of information in about one minute.
-   Using highly technical terms, acronyms or slangs. You want your pitch to be easily understood. Avoid using words that will confuse the average person. The last thing you want is that, whoever is listening to you, feels dumb.
-   Not being focused. This isn't a general conversation, you're not discussing the weather. Keep your pitch clear

and focused. Focus on what you do.

- Not practicing. First, write down your pitch. Read it over. Have your friends and family read it. Does it make sense? Make sure it flows well and that there aren't any spots that feel rough or awkward. Then practice it, practice it again. Keep practicing it until it becomes so easy for you to pitch that.
- Being too robotic. This is all about a face to face interaction with someone you want to impress. Look for an easily approachable compensation style for your pitch.
- Not having a business card or other takeaway with you. Imagine you've sold them on you. They are convinced. Now how are they going to get a hold of you when they decide it's time to go into your office? Make sure you always have something on you to pass on that will allow people to not only remember you but contact you later.

Template for your Elevator Pitch

Hi, my name is Peter Smith

I am a smile creating dentist,

helping people who are unhappy with
the appearance of their teeth

My greatest passion is to design and build
the exclusive smiles of their dreams they love
and enjoy

I´ve been fortunate to have gone through
years of training in esthetic dentistry and
dental implants to be able to help over 5000 patients
from all over the world to smile again

have you ever thought about enhancing your smile?

10
PERSONAL BRANDING SECRETS

Here you will learn in what areas you can increase your brand and how to increase that brand. You will get an action plan for your personal branding and free tools to scan your personal brand.

Again, what's branding? Branding is influencing. It is an enduring perception of you. You project your brand to others.

What others think about you, that's your brand.

Elements that help you in your branding would be patient testimonials. You should ask for a personal testimonial. If they are happy, they should give you a testimonial.

And even better if this testimonial is done in videos. If you have a video, you can take the text of that video and just publish it as a text. You can take the sound of the video and publish it as a sound, and you can take the whole video, you can take pictures of that video. This gives you a variety of possibilities to take advantage of that testimonial. If you have a video wall or something like that on in your office, you can put the patient in front of it with your logo on the back and then just take your mobile phone and let the patient speak about his experience.

Thank-you letters are also very good to publish. Also emails.

Networking: you should network in your community. You should make social engagements in your community. This helps to build your brand, because people think of you not only as a dentist, also as a person that is engaged in the community, a person, who is helping others in the community. This will make your brand bigger.

Your business cards: just let them move.

Joint ventures with hairdressers or beauty salons. if you can partner up with them, that you send them your patients and they send you their clients. This would be awesome for your brand, but look always at the top three of your city and partner only with them.

Physicians, physical therapists and always the top ones in town.

You should give seminars, a presentation workshop. In schools, in pharmacies, in health clubs. 30 minutes maximum. I have had the experience, that people are focused 20 to 30 minutes and after that it is too long-lasting. Make it short. Make it 30 minutes.

Talk about a topic. Like 'Questions you have about dental implants' or 'How to effectively get rid of bad breath', something like that. You can prepare that in 30 or 20 minutes and then leave 10 minutes for questions, done. Take a lot of business cards with you.

Public relations: you should prepare a media kit with CV, photos and a resume and send it to everybody that is asking for information about you, like the press and all the media.

Also put in the links to press and media releases, that are already out there, so that they can have a look at them.

Internet, videos, social media: build an email list that with people, that subscribe to your list. You can use free services for that, like mailerlite.com.

The more videos you have, the bigger your brand is. The more content you publish on social media, the bigger your brand is.

An action plan for your personal brand, what should you do?

You should give two interviews per month on either local TV, radio, podcast, press, or similar. If you don't have media, that want to publish the interview about you, then you just make up an interview yourself and you publish it somewhere in free areas or websites, that publish external links. And then you have an interview published.

Make one video every week on a dental topic.

There are so many dental topics. Every question you get through email, you can make a video about that. Every question you hygienists get from the patient, you can make a video about that. Every question a patient asked at the reception, you can make a video about that. And maybe about organizational items, things about your office and how to make an appointment or things like that. It doesn't have to be only strictly about teeth.

Make one presentation a month in pharmacies, in health clubs, in schools. Publish every day in your social media.

Action Plan for your Personal Branding

Give 2 interviews per month (local TV, Radio, Podcast, Press)
Make 1 video every week on a dental topic
make 1 presentation a month
publish every day in your social media

Free tools for monitoring your personal brand online

reputation: google.com/alerts. It updates every day. And it's better if you search with quotations like "your office" or "your name".

Then you can see whatever is published about you.

Everybody's talking about you. Socialmentions.com is the same thing,
but for social media.

tineye.com. That's pictures of you, that are somewhere else or that are moving around the internet, maybe something you don't like maybe something you like. So you can see, who uses your images.

11
BE THE EXPERT FOR YOUR DENTAL PATIENTS

This chapter is about how to be the expert for your patients. You have to specialize, be the expert is to be specialized in something. Something like in invisible orthodontics or, in veneers, in smile design, in sleep apnea, sleep dentistry and the list can go on.

Specialize not only in dentistry also in your patients. You have to specialize in certain patients. For example, wealthy patients, wealthy over 40 years.

So you carefully choose a target market and then develop your treatments to meet their needs. What do these people need? If everyone is your patient Nobody is your patient. That's very sad, but it's true.

Choose who you want to treat, and then cater to them. Your marketing and branding should exclude any other possible patient. Exclude them, so that your message is not attractive to them. That is better than to say: don't come.

Your sales should be inclusive, your marketing should be exclusive. Once your wanted patient is in your office, your communication should really help him to go for the treatment, that you want him to do.

The more often you reject the patients you don't really want, the more you attract the patients that you really want.

Don't wait for permission. Claim the expert position and then back it up. If you wait until you really are considered the expert, a lot of time goes by. You can claim to be the expert in XYZ. You claim it and then you show that you really are the expert in that, so that everybody will look at you as an expert in that field.

Ways to specialize, for example, are
- by ability, you have a better ability or greater results? You can show them, prove them, then you are specialized in that special treatment where you get better results or you are really very good at. It is difficult to prove. Maybe you got some awards, or some testimonials of patients that back you up, and that can show, that you have that special ability in these kinds of treatments.
- Maybe your treatments are faster.
- In some of the treatments, you're so good that you can give a really long guarantee.
- Or you open a wide range of treatments, that are focused on the patients, that you want to attract into your office.
- By education, you get some postgraduate studies and you have a diploma. So you can show: I'm an expert in this area.
- By mission: showing your objectives. That your objectives are different than the objectives of other dentists. Look for the chapter about mission and vision statement that I wrote. And you specialize in a special field of dentistry only by your vision statement.
- By attribute: any characteristic, that is attractive or beneficial for your target patient, for example, personality type, age, skill, education interests, maybe your wealthy patients want you to be a Ph.D., well, then you make a Ph.D. Maybe your target patients want you also to be a

little bit older, because they fear that young dentists cannot have the skills they want. Then you have to appear older, if you're not older, you behave older, you dress older, you grow a beard so that you appear older. If your target audience wants that, if not, no problem.

How do you know your target audience wants something? You subscribe to journals or to online journals your target audience is interested in.

For example, if you want to attract wealthy people, then the ROBB report would be a good choice for you. There you see what's the interest and then you assimilate these interests and you cater later to them.

Now you have to ask yourself, what do you want to be known for? And what do you want to be known as? I want to be known for doing this and that. I want to be known as the best dentist in town, the best dentist in invisible orthodontics or whatever. These are your aims, and then try to get your ideal patient in with your goal settings.

Key elements of an effective personal brand:

-   Your backstory. What's your story? Tell stories, tell people how you did it, how you made it, what you went through to be where you are now. You might say to yourself, that a lot of dentists went through the same experiences as well. So what, you tell your story. And patients love that.
-   What you stand for, your beliefs, your values. Transmit them, make videos with that, make publications with that, put it on your website.
-   Your superpower: one ability, that you have, that you think you're very good in. Magnify it, make it big, make it all turn around it. That means all your communication will turn around this idea, but you have to be good at

that, really good.

- And if you're good at nothing, you go to a post-graduate program or workshop and you learn one thing. And this one thing you learn really good, from a person that is really showing how it's done.
- Your stories: marketing is storytelling. People love stories. Just put your story together. That's your backstory what you stand for, your superpower.
- Insider language. You can say I'm an expert in XYZ, and you come up with something. I'm the first doing this or that. It might be a cleaning, normal cleaning, but you change a little bit on the cleaning and then you are first in town or the first in the country to do that type of cleaning.
- Make acronyms out of this. Apart of that modified cleaning for example. First expert in the B.E.S.T.-technique. And B.E.S.T. could stand for: Beauty Enhancing Smile Treatment. That's a smile design you might say. Yes, I know. And I'm not the first one to make a smile design, you might say. I know, but you're the very first in doing the B.E.S.T.-technique in smile design. You came up with it, okay? It is not a very good example but I think you get the idea. Come up with your own ideas in your field.

ABOUT MARKETING

12
WHY AND HOW DENTISTS SHOULD DO VIDEO MARKETING

In this chapter I will write about why and how dentists should do video marketing.

You will learn why it is better than other methods and marketing strategies, how to structure an up to 10 minutes video, when to upload it, and how to structure a YouTube video ad and how to find a good title for your video.

Video marketing is attraction marketing. But there are other types of marketing like interruption marketing, in the malls.

Interruption marketing: When you go to a mall and there is a booth with credit cards or so and they stop you. You're going to go somewhere else but they stop you and they ask you: do you have a credit card? And that is annoying.

Also in Facebook you find interruption marketing: the sponsored ads. You are reading the posts of your friends and families, and of the groups you are in, and all of a sudden there are some sponsored ads. That's annoying.

Attraction marketing is when someone is looking up something, and your video comes up on YouTube or Google or somewhere else.

Here's a template for a 10 minutes video.

- Start. The first five seconds is all about grabbing attention maybe with a question. You have to say: Hey, I'm here. That's grabbing attention.

- The next 10 to 15 seconds is to introduce yourself and reveal the main benefits of the video. Why should they watch this video?

- and then you should make an opener logo like 10 to 15 seconds. For example, you can go to the websites of videohive.net for some introduction videos, you just put in your logo into that and in audiojungle.net is for music that you can buy and then put it as background for this logo-introduction-video.

- After that, the main content, it's two to seven minutes. It depends on what content you want to show. You want to show how to brush your teeth, you brush your teeth. You want to show how to floss, you show that. You want to show how to scrape your tongue or how is the experience the first time a patient comes to the office? You make a video about that.

- Then, in the end, you have to have a call to action. Maybe one, that people should subscribe to your channel, watch more videos, ask questions or they should call a number and come to your office or visit your website. What do you want people to do after they watch the video?

- Then the final exit video. Listing your social media or

something like that. You can also go to videohive and look for templates of that to upload.

Statistics have shown, that the best time to upload a video is Tuesdays at 9 am.

The second choice would be Thursdays the same time.

The third best option is Wednesdays or Fridays also the same time.

Here's a template for video for a YouTube ad.
- The first five seconds you grab attention maybe with a question,

- then you talk about the pain points, their struggle and talk about feelings on how you will make them feel. How good they feel before the treatment and after the treatment.

- And the solution. You try to give them a view on the solution. You show them, that you have the solution for the bad feelings they are in now (either real, or provoked by putting a seed in their mind with your question at the beginning) and how they get to the good feeling after the treatment. This treatment helps you to do this and that or to have this and that. For example, this periodontal treatment helps you to get rid of your bleeding in the gums and to have fresh breath. Or to get rid of your pain, if the pain point is bad breath.

- Then a call to action. What do you want people to do after they watch the video?

- And then final exit video, social media like 10 seconds to show, that you are on social media, that you have a Facebook site, that you have a web page, and so on.

Tips on how to find a good title for your video. Like for advertisements, you have to have the same strategy.

- Stated as a question. Do you want to...? or Would you like to...? Do you want to learn how to brush your teeth thoroughly? or Do you want to know how the first-time experience in our office is? Would you like to see a patient's experience the first time he comes into our office?

- State it as a secret. For example: Secrets on how to get rid of snoring at night. Then you can talk about all your sleep dentistry devices or treatments.

- Make it newsy. Introducing, announcing, discover. For example, Announcing the new ceramic dental implants. Then you talk about new implants you've bought and how you will put them into the patients.

13
TIPS ON HOW TO HANDLE MEDIA AND PRESS

In this chapter, we want to talk about tips on how to handle the media and press. You will learn where to find help. You will learn how to handle TV interviews. What is bridging during an interview, on TV, or even radio? How to prepare the interview, an interview checklist, how to handle radio interviews, and how to handle press interviews.

The first step is to hire a publicist. A publicist is a person whose job is to generate and manage publicity for a company, brand or public figure.

Most top-level publicists work in private practice handling multiple clients. Usually, they are journalists and they can have so many contacts in media and press, that they make you newsworthy.

You will not pay to get into the media, into TV, into radio, into press. You don't pay to the media. It is not paid advertisement, which always looks fake and is suspicious. So, it's not advertisement. You pay this publicist for his service. That's the idea.

Find a good one, and if you don't have the money to pay that publicist, try to trade your service against his service, bleachings, veneers, ortho-treatment. For him, for his family. If he refuses, find one who is open to that idea. This is a tip for the case, that you would not have the money to pay the publicist.

Television

For television interviews, you need to prepare the issue, of course. They will probably tell you, that they will talk about this or that actor, because something special is in their teeth or they had a makeover or they have a diastema, or a crown fell off in an interview. Or they want to talk about the grills, that are now on vogue.

You should prepare that. You have to research, you have to talk to dental technicians about it, how they handle that, in case you have not made a grill before. You just gather information about grills, for example.

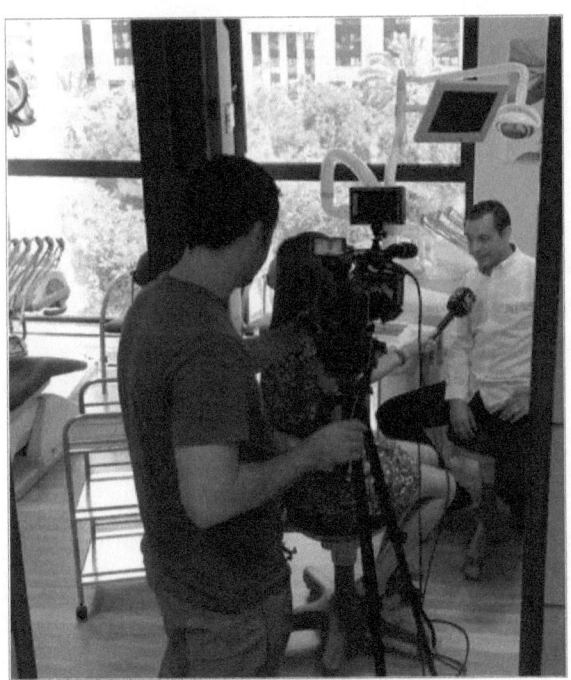

Assume what you say before the actual interview will also be used. So, whatever you tell the journalist before the camera is on, this will also be used, or it could be used. So be careful what you say. For example, if you say: I don't believe in grills, but as I am here, I will talk about grills. So be careful.

Be credible, talk credible, look credible.

Be short, concise and to the point in the answers. They love, short and precise answers.

Bridging

Bridging is when you don't want to answer a question. Imagine there is a question that you don't want to answer or you want to get your (a different) message across. The conversation or the questions are going into a direction, that is not your direction.
And you want to redirect this conversation or these questions. Then you bridge.
You start with a phrase that helps you to go in your direction. What is that phrase? There are different options of doing that, for example:
- Yes, I have heard that and what I can tell you…. and you start to go into your direction about it.
- This is not scientifically proven at the moment, and what I can tell you….. and then you continue.
- Before I answer that question, can I just give you some background information …… and then your information, your message is that background information.
- I prefer to look at it this way…… and then you get your message across.

Learn these sentences and use them if you want to redirect the conversation.

What you don't have to do:
- don't use contradicting information.
- Don't use technical words. That sounds too arrogant.
- Don't use notes. Don't look at the notes the whole time when you talk.
- Don't talk fast.
- Don't talk bad about others.
- Don't get angry.
- Don't be like a statue.

A trick is to use your hands. Sometimes you just explain things better with your hands.

Television can come to your office, or you can be invited to a plateau. And it's the same thing. Usually the same questions arise.

Interview checklist.

Preparation will help you control the interview. The interview will be conducted randomly. The media loves controversy. They want a good story. So, they will ask questions that are a little be tricky sometimes. But you can give them a good story and at the same time, get what you want.

You want to promote yourself. That's the idea of being there.

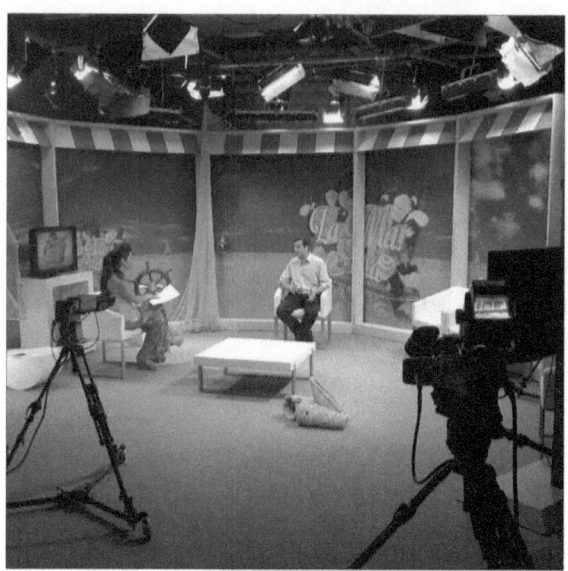

Prepare these questions about your topic veneers, grills or whatever is the topic:
- You think about the most damaging question. Like, do grills damage the teeth? Something like that or do veneers damage teeth? or does bleaching damage teeth?
- The most challenging question. That is a little bit more scientific, more high level.
- A subject to avoid and the reason. If that question comes up, you say: I better will not talk about this because of that and that, and then you prepare bridging sentences.
- The most researched question.
- The most logical question.
- The most intelligent question.
- The most difficult question.
- The most delicate question.
- The most controversial question.

Think about all these questions, prepare them, and then you have a good set of questions, that could come from the interviewer.

Of course, if the interviewer gives you already the list of questions, that he or she prepared, it's easy for you. Just prepare these questions. But with this checklist, you are not only prepared for the questions, you also are preparing your answers to these questions.

Remember, it should be short and precise and to the point.

Radio

In radio it is very similar. For radio interviews, prepare the issue better.

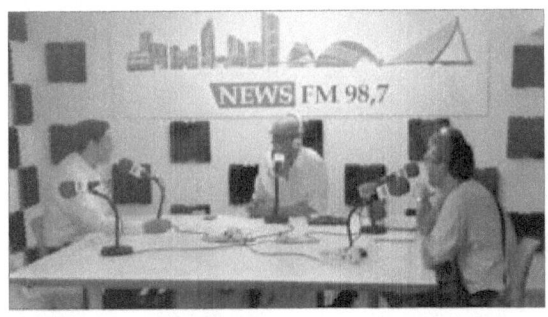

It's better in the studio than over the phone. So, if they call you and they say: we want to make an interview with you, would you come to the studio or should we call you on the phone? It's better in the studio.

Why? Because you see the interviewer and you can interact better. You can create a pleasant atmosphere before the interview. And everybody is happier. You can look the people that ask you the questions into the eyes, and explain as if you would explain it directly to him.

Take paper and pencil with you. Maybe they don't have that (they usually have it).

Have a smile in your voice. Assume the microphone is always on. That means, that if you say something that is outside of the interview, think that it could be recorded. Think that it could be aired.

Speak clearly and slowly.

Call the host by his or her name. That's very important. They like that, and then their attitude is very positive towards you, and they will invite you again.

The don'ts: they are more or less the same as on TV.
- Don't use contradicting information.
- Don't use technical words. They sound arrogant.
- Don't react to negative energy of negative callers if they call into the studio or the radio program. If they are negative, don't react to that negativity. Don't be negative yourself.
- Don't talk fast.
- Don't talk bad about others.
- Don't get angry.

<u>Press</u>

In printed media, they usually send the interview to you per email, or they call you per phone, or the reporter comes to your office. In these cases everything you say can be printed.

Try to find out the questions beforehand and prepare for them.

Usually the print-media ask many more questions than the radio or the TV reporter.

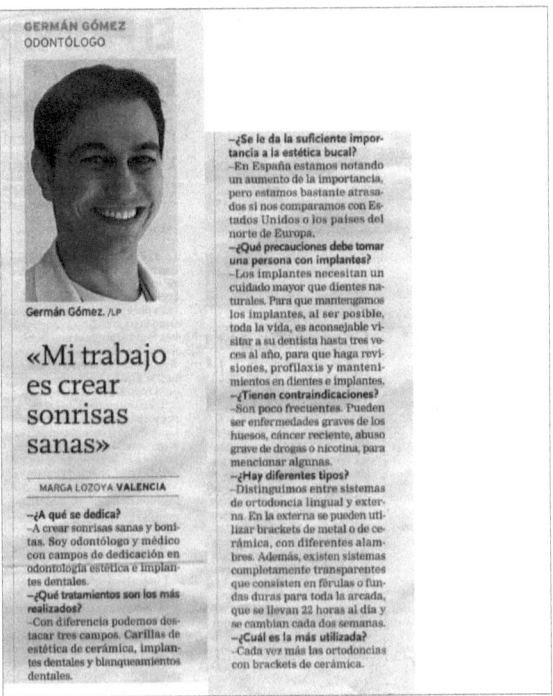

Dress appropriately. They might want to take pictures. Don't think, "it's the press. I don't need to look good".

And you come in like, not shaved, because that day you don't see patients. They can suddenly say, let's make a picture and then you look like an amateur. So be dressed appropriately and look smart.

And make at least 10 interviews per year. This will boost you!

14
HOW TO STIMULATE REFERRALS

We will talk about how to stimulate referrals, what usually happens, and you some strategies to increase referrals and how to handle a "no" if somebody doesn't want to refer to you.

What usually happens is, this: When you ask dentists, where most of their business comes from, they usually answer, that it's from referrals.

But most dentist's strategy is this: First, they hope, but hope is not a strategy. They hope, that people will talk about them, and people will refer to them.

Second, they might ask: "if you know somebody who needs my dentistry, please let me know". This is what they usually say to the patients. In this case there is an action, which is good. But if the patient says, "I don't know anybody right now". Then what happens next? Nothing happens, nothing fast and continuous happens.

What strategies should you have?

Strategy number one:
Avoid the word referral when you are asking for referrals. Instead of using the word "referrals" use the word "introduce". "Could you think of some friends, colleagues or family that you could introduce to me?".

Strategy number two:
Ask for permission before you even treat them. The first time the patient comes in, you set the expectations. Your expectation is, that this patient as a new patient will refer to you patients later on. You can say that from the beginning of the relationship. "Mr. patient, my purpose is to help you to become so happy with the treatment, that you gladly would introduce me to at least three people you really care about" or "Mr. patient, I want you to be so delighted with the treatment, that at the end, I will ask you to introduce me to at least three people you really care about, does that seem fair enough?".

And then he knows, that you will do anything possible to make him happy, which is good. And in return, he gives you referrals. Of course, you would have tried to make him happy anyhow, but now he feels like he needs to give you something in return.

Now you have set the tone.

Strategy number three:
Imagine you have asked for advice instead of referrals. Imagine you have a highly successful patient. And you want more of these celebrities, soccer players, american football players or basketball players or something like that.

Sometimes they're not comfortable being mentioned. They don't want you to mention them, because they have contracts with advertisement companies. It happens to me a lot, by the way.

So, what do you do? If you ask directly, they feel uncomfortable, they don't like that usually. You have to apply another strategy.

You ask for advice in three steps.

Step number one: acknowledgment. What does that mean? "Mr. patient, I want to sincerely thank you for your confidence in us to help you design your new smile. And I'm truly grateful.". You acknowledge a patient for being your patient and for his confidence.

Step number two: put him or her in your place. "Imagine you were me and run a dental office and you want to help more people like you, highly successful patients. And you would love to work with people who are introduced by good patients."

Step number three: ask for advice. "I'm curious what would a successful person like you do, to encourage people like you to introduce your friends, colleagues and families to a dentist like me?".

These are highly successful people. They will come with ideas on the spot so you just have to implement these ideas. And then you do it on them. So now it is difficult for them not to introduce you to their environment because it was *their* idea to proceed the way you're proceeding on them at that moment.

They gave you a tip on how to proceed, and you do it on them. Does it work? They told you, that this would work, so then they would have to refer patients to you.

Strategy number four:
What if the patient says "no, I don't want to refer". Find out what has happened, and what has to happen. "Mr. patient, I would love to be the person who you would feel comfortable introducing to your friends and family". Notice, we do not use the word refer. We use "introduce".

"Let me ask you a question. What should happen now, in order to make that a reality?" Take notes and let them talk. What has to happen?

Then "Mr. patient, let's pretend I do ABC, that you suggest. Would you be more comfortable to introduce two or three of your friends to us?" "Sure". That's it, you got it.

That's how you get referrals.

You don't hope you don't wait.

You proactively use words you use a script, the scripts in the strategies, that I just presented to you.

15
PATIENT REFERRAL SCRIPT
STEP-BY-STEP

In this chapter, we will talk about how to ask for patient referrals, an example script step by step.

You will learn when the best time is to ask for a referral.

How to ask for a referral. What words to use and why.

And all this inside of a step by step script. It's an example script. It's not the best script ever, but it has helped me in a certain way.

Everybody agrees, that they want more referrals. But nearly no dentist really asks for a referral. So why do they do that? Why don't they ask for that?

There are five main reasons.

First of all, they are too afraid to ask. Don't be too afraid. If you don't ask you don't get one. But if you want some, you have to ask. There is nothing to be afraid of, when you believe, that your work and your service are good. If you don't believe that, you have to improve it, and then ask for referrals.

Second: they are too lazy. I don't think a lot of dentists are really too lazy to do that. You are reading this book, Laziness is not one of your characteristics. So let's move to the next possible reason.

Third: they are too proud. Some might think: "I am a dentist or physician. I don't want to give the impression, that I beg the patient for a referral." It's not true.

You are giving a compliment to the patient because you tell the patient, that you want more people like him in your office. That's good for him, because you say it's positive to have him in your office. It is empowering. You don't have to be too proud. You don't seem needy or begging. That's completely untrue.

Forth: they don't know when to ask.

When somebody is happy and shows gratitude. You have to wait for these two words: If these two words come up, then is the time for you to ask for a referral. The two words are, "thank you".

If the patient says thank you. He shows gratitude. Not only "Thanks". Thank you!

If you hear these two words, then is the time to say: "Now I will ask".

Fifth: they don't know how to ask.

You start with a question. You have to make people agree to an action, before they know what action you will ask them to do. You have to make your patient agree to give you a referral, before he even knows, that you will ask him for a referral. How is that possible?

You use these words: "You couldn't do me a small favor, could you?"

So, the patient says thank you.

You say: you couldn't do me a small favor, could you?

Then he says, Well, I guess or It depends.

The human body and the human brain are programmed for this: if somebody asks for a favor, it immediately has the reflex to respond with Yes, but some people have a certain limit to that and say: well it depends.

But nobody will say "no" immediately.

It depends on whether or not he can do what you will ask him to do. Or whether or not it is easy to do or difficult to do.

So, if you give him an action, that is easy to do, he will do it.

Then you tell them what the action it is he has to take: "You wouldn't happen to know..." Notice, we use these words instead of "Do you know somebody?". You don't say that. Instead you say "you wouldn't happen to know".

Because if you say it this way it's like a challenge. You suggest with this, that he probably won't. But it would be cool if he would.

Now immediately the brain of the patient starts to be motivated and starts to search.

Next step: "You wouldn't happen to know..... just one person.". You narrow it down to just one person. You make it really easy for the patient to search. To do what you want him to do. Instead of "somebody" you say "just one person".

"Somebody" would have the most of the time as a result, that the patient says, that he would come back to you with the suggestion. If you say "somebody" he usually answers: "I will think about somebody and I come back to you". By the way, they never come back to us.

So, it is better to say "You wouldn't happen to know just one person". This is more a more reasonable request and you concentrate his mind's effort and make it easy for him.

Then you continue.

"You wouldn't happen to know just one person…. who just like you, would benefit from…." and then you put in what you want to sell. Like implants, if you did implants on him.

"You wouldn't happen to know just one person, who, just like you, would benefit from implants" or from a smile-makeover or a smile design or veneers or from whatever you want. Periodontal treatment or prophylaxis. Whatever you've done to the patient, and he's grateful for.

You just throw that line after you have asked for a favor a small favor.

This helps them to choose that person.

Then you shut up. Don't say anything.

The patient starts to think. Let him think. So they start to think, they start to move, thinking, moving, crossing the arms, thinking. And then, all of a sudden, his physiognomy changes. The expression changes.

Then is the time they have found someone. They have found the name of someone, but maybe they are not very confident. They are uncomfortable to tell you the name because they don't want to compromise that person.

In this moment, when they change their expression and their body language, you say, to calm this uncomfortable feeling down:

"don't worry….". The patient changes again his expression towards a more relaxed one.

"I'm not looking for the details *right now*, but who is it that you're thinking of?". And then he tells you the name, relaxed, only the name. "It's John",

Then you have two versions to continue:

Version A:
"Great. When are you going to next speak to John?"
They say, "Saturday", for example.
Then you say: "Great. Couldn't you do me a further favor?
Could you? When you speak to John, wouldn't you mind having
a short conversation about your experience in our office?"
"Sure."
You continue: "And see if he is open-minded to call us to see
if we can help him the same way we helped you?"

I repeat that again.
"Great. you couldn't do me another favor, could you? When
you speak to John. wouldn't you mind having a short
conversation about your experience in our office and see if he's
open-minded to call us to see if we can help him the same way
we have helped you?"
So there, you're giving him exactly directions on when to ask
his prospect or his friend or his colleague and when to tell him
about us and what to do.

So, you did with this script, several things:
-   you chose the time you told the patient to give you a
    referral.
-   You made him think about somebody
-   and find somebody
-   and then you gave instructions on when to talk to him
-   and how to talk to him.
-   A short conversation about your experience in our office,
    and see if he's open-minded. So telling him about that
    and then asking him if he could call us.
-   And you give the patient your business card to give that
    to the possible patient.

You could stop here and then wait for the possible patient to call you. But if you want to take it to a further level of control, you have the:

Version B:
This version starts the same way
"Great. When are you going to next speak to John?"
They say, "Saturday", for example.
Then you say: "Great. Couldn't you do me a further favor? Could you?
When you speak to John, wouldn't you mind having a short conversation about your experience in our office?"
"Sure."
You continue: "And see if he is open-minded *to take a call from me* to see if we can help him the same way we helped you?"

So in this version you call this friend or colleague or relative. But in order to call him, you have to start to follow up to get the information of that other possible patient.

You have to find out whether or not this possible patient told him, that you could call him. What you say is:

"When can I call you quickly to find out how your chat with John went?". So, if it was supposed to be on Saturday, you say,

"Would Monday or Tuesday be okay for you?". You give two options.

He says "Yes Monday". Then you say:
"Monday morning or afternoon?"
He answers maybe: "afternoon".
"3 pm would be okay?".
"Yes, sure."
"Good."

And then you have to call. You write down when you have to call, so you don't forget it, and you call.
When you call, you say these words:

"I'm just calling as promised." This means you are a man or a woman of your word.

They might reply with "Thank you".

Then you take the tension out of your patient. He could have talked to his friend or not. The best is you already assume he did not. You say this:

"I'm guessing you didn't get around to speak to John.". Now there are two options. He did or he did not.

If he did, he will say: "I did. He's happy to hear from you. Here are the details." Or "he's not happy to hear from you. or he's not open-minded.".

In this case you say: "Could you think about one other person?" And you go through the whole process again.

Option 2: "Oh, I forgot. But I call him today or tomorrow."
At least you accelerate with your call that possibility.

Let's go over the script again.

When? When you hear "Thank you"

How? First with a question:
"You couldn't do me a small favor, could you?"
"sure"
"You wouldn't happen to know, just one person who, like you, would benefit from veneers?"
Then shut up.
When they change their expression, when they found somebody,
then you say:
"Don't worry."
They relax.
"I'm not looking for the details right now. But who is it that you're thinking of?"
They say the name

"Great. When are you going to next speak to *name*?"

"Saturday."

"Great. You couldn't do me a further favor, could you? When you speak to *name*, wouldn't you mind having a short conversation about the experience in our office and see if he's open-minded to call us to see if we can help him the same way we helped you?"

That's one version.

The other version is:

"...and see if he's open-minded to take a call from me to see if we can help him the same way we have helped you?"

If you choose the other version, then you have to continue.

"When can I call you quickly to find out how your chat with *name* went? Would Monday or Tuesday be okay?"

Then you set the time and you call that day.

"I'm just calling as promised."

"I'm guessing you didn't get around to speak to *name*?"

and then they tell you what, what's going on.

ABOUT THE SALES PROCESS

16
5 REASONS PATIENTS
DON'T BUY YOUR TREATMENTS

This chapter will talk about five reasons patients don't buy your treatments and how to react to these situations, and how to make your case acceptance more successful.

<u>Reason number one.</u>

No need or low need at that moment.
You should explain to them why their health needs the treatment if they don't see the need. You need to make them see that need.

If you fail in that, then it's better to save time and move on and try maybe in a year or so. In this case follow up in half a year or in a year.

But the main thing is, you need them to recognize and to see the need in that treatment.

<u>Reason number two.</u>

There is no urgency. Delay kills the sale! If they come up with "Maybe in a month, in two months, maybe later I will do that treatment", this means, that it will not happen.

It's either now or it will not happen. Show why it should be done right now. Maybe you come up with an exclusive offer, an offer you do only right now at that moment, not later. And that's why they should do it right now.

For example, you bought 10 bleaching kits for a very, very good price. And you tell the patient "Listen, I've bought 10 bleaching kits for a really good price. And I can make a good offer on the bleaching right now, because there is only a limited quantity of 10. And you can get one of these for a special price", for example.

That is how you create urgency. There are ways to create urgency. Try to give them a push. It is like giving them a small reason, why they should do it right now.

So, reason number two was no urgency, you have to create urgency by exclusive offers or limited quantity. That's urgency.

<u>Reason number three.</u>

No desire. People usually don't buy what they need, or what is the right thing to do. Maybe *you* are convinced he needs the treatment, a periodontal treatment, for example, but the patient is not convinced. He doesn't see the need, or if he sees the need, he doesn't want it.

People do not always want what they need. They buy what they want! For example, they want the new Michael Kors™ bag or shoes or a vacation.

Do they really need that bag? These shoes, that vacation? No, they don't, they don't need that. They might need much, much more a periodontal treatment or an implant or whatever you suggest. But they don't want it.

They want that vacation. They want that Michael Kors™ bag. We don't actually need a lot of things, but we want them. We have the desire.

Here is a way you have to create the desire. With an irresistible offer, for example. Or you highlight the existing desires, they already have, and connect them to the treatment.

For example, veneers. Veneers can make the social acceptance of that person much better. They are more likable.

People want to be likable.

People want to be attractive.

People want to be confident.

People want to be socially accepted.

You have to relate your treatment, to that desire. Like a missing tooth, for example, doesn't make you very attractive, doesn't make you smile with confidence. That is why you need an implant.

You see the difference? They do not need an implant. They need to be socially accepted. They need to be attractive. They need to be confident.

This is what you have to aim at in your argumentation. Not that they need an implant. This is something they don't want, but they want to be socially accepted. They want to be attractive and they want to be confident.

Reason number four.

No money. They don't have the money. They don't have a budget, but who has a yearly planned budget for dentistry? People usually have a budget for a vacation, they have a budget for Christmas gifts and so on. We have a budget for our car and so on.

But who has a budget for dentistry? Who has reserved money for dentistry? Literally nobody.

So, they don't have a budget. What's new about that? They don't have the money now available. That usually means they don't see the value in your treatment.

They don't see why that costs so much. If they don't see the value, we haven't presented the benefits of the treatment the way, that the value is higher than the price. A high value is exactly what I was addressing before. Valuable for the patients means social acceptance, it means being attractive, it means being confident. That has a high value for the patient.

The higher the value the less the price is important. If you can create in the patient's mind the picture, that the treatment has a high value for them, then the price is not so important. They will find the money to pay for it.

And if they don't find the money, why don't you put some financing options together? Talk to your bank, if they can finance small treatments for your patients. Talk to third parties, that offer financial services to give you different options.

Reason number five.

No trust. They just don't trust you. Give them more social proof. Like testimonials, like before and afters. Have your own cases. Show them, and tell stories about the patients. "This patient was just like you. And here's how he or she looked like after the treatment. You see how confident she smiles? See how beautiful she is."

Attractiveness, confidence, social acceptance, social proof.

Tell them your background, make sure they know.

I did that postgraduate program,

I graduated in this university,

I have so many years of experience all these things.

You have to make them know. How do you make them know? By telling them why you treat them, by making your hygienist tell them why she's doing the cleaning.

This gives them more reasons to trust you.

Sometimes they doubt about themselves and not you. That means they think it will not work for them. It's a waste of money. For example, the last bridge they had failed, why should it be different with you, you have to give them reasons for that, for example: "We are using so zirconium, this kind of bridges are very new and they don't fail like the ones, that have been put on you last time". "In your case, this is the correct decision", or: "in this case, we include one more pillar, one more tooth to make it more stable". This is one reason.

The other thing is, you tell them that you put them in a hygiene program to increase success in the long term. They're not left alone. "Once we do that bridge, once we do that treatment, you get into our recall-hygiene program. You come in every six months, we check, we maintain, so that we make this a success on the long term. This treatment should be a success in a long term. You are not left alone. We are here to maintain this treatment."

This is the kind of message you should transmit to the patient. This is something you have to tell them. And remember:

No need, no sale.
No urgency, no sale.
No desire, no sale.
No money, no sale
and no trust, no sale.

17
5 MISTAKES DENTISTS MAKE
WHEN THEY TRY TO SELL TREATMENTS

In this chapter, I want to talk to you about the five mistakes dentists make when they try to sell treatments.

First of all, we have to make clear that the decision of the patient is based on trust and only trust. If they trust us, they will make the treatment with us.

Mistake number one.

Trying to sell a premium treatment at a low price.

You try to sell something really valuable, really high end, really a lot of work, high-quality materials, high-quality treatment at a low price.

First of all, people start to be skeptical and they will think, that it cannot be true. Because their perception is, when your service is offered at a low price, that this is a cheap treatment. They don't value really what you do for them, you do a really good treatment for a low price.

They don't see it like a really good treatment, they see it as a cheap treatment at a cheap price.

<u>Mistake number two.</u>

Selling a low-value treatment to a premium patient.

Premium patients. These patients buy based on emotions and feelings. They do not buy based on price. That's why you will not have a good result.

Imagine a Rolex™ offer: buy one, get one free. Or a 40% discount before this deadline. This will not happen with Rolex™. Rolex™ is selling to a premium customer. As you are selling in this moment to a premium patient, you should not make a low-value treatment or a low-value offer or cheap offer.

<u>Mistake number three.</u>

Trying to sell a high-value treatment in a low value setting.

The environment is important. If the environment is okay, then trust in that treatment is all right. If you go to a restaurant and the burger is €5 and the chicken fingers for €6, and all of a sudden on the menu, there appears a premium steak for €120. The client will think, that there is something wrong. In this case you expect something more around 20 to €30 a steak. But €5 a burger, €6 chicken fingers and a premium steak €120? This is not the place for it.

You have to ask yourself: is your office the place for a high-value treatment? If yes, offer it, if not, transform your office into a place for a high-value treatment. Do not offer it in a low value setting.

If the fillings are €40 it's infinitely more difficult to sell a full smile-makeover for 15,000 or €20,000.

If you already have high prices for bleaching, for fillings, for cleanings, then everybody expects the smile-makeover not to be cheap. The environment is important.

Mistake number four.

Trying to sell a high-value treatment to low-value patients.

Nobody will buy that treatment. Why? Because this kind of patients don't appreciate the value of what you are offering. They are looking for cheap things.

And because they don't buy, you start to question your offer and you think: "oh, maybe the price is too high". No, it's not too high. You're trying to sell that to the wrong people. That's the problem.

You think it does not work? It will work. You only have to offer that to the correct people.

Mistake number five.

Trying to sell a high-value treatment with a low-value mindset.

Your confidence and belief in the value is important. If you really believe, that what you do has a high value, and what you do has the highest possible quality, then charge the highest possible prices for it.

It is more about yourself. It is more about the fear in you to set the price too high. Maybe in the beginning, you are not comfortable. Maybe you have to watch your body language because maybe your lips say "this is a high-value offer. I make this make-over for 20,000 euros", but your body language is like, "maybe it's too expensive".

Your body language has to show that you're very confident with that price that you're very confident with the quality that you offer. That's why you have to watch your body language.

Say the high price as if it was no big deal. Maybe you have to practice it. You practice it over and over again, so that it is very fluent, and very normal for you to say the high price.

Watch your language. What do you say? How do you say it?

And remember: all price resistance is in you, not in the patient. You set the price and it's your resistance to set a high price. Do not make resistance against yourself.

18
A SIMPLE IDEA ON HOW TO
HANDLE OBJECTIONS

In this chapter, we will talk about a simple idea on how to handle objections. It is based on the simple three F idea to follow. You just have to follow these three steps, that are based on three F's. And you can do that every time a patient comes up with any objection. It is very simple.

When a patient comes up with an objection, this is a resistance he is applying. The patient builds up resistance against your offer, your treatment plan, your suggestion.

He is giving you all kinds of objections, doesn't matter what kind of objection, it is an objection.

You need to redirect this energy to get to the close. With this three F method. And here is how it works:

The first F is feel.

Step one, you have to show empathy. But not just fake empathy, but real empathy. You have to understand this objection.

Do not push against the objection. Do not fight it. Don't argue. Instead, try to say this:

"You know what? I understand how you feel". Or "I can see where you're coming from. I understand". You don't have to necessarily use the word feel. Or just "I understand, Yes". Something like that. You have to show real empathy.

<u>The second F is felt.</u>

Step two, let the patient see he is not alone.
"Other patients felt the same way". Or "I felt the same way".
A lot of people have felt the same way, have thought the same way, or had the same problem.

<u>The third F is found.</u>

Step three, show them the solution. "Here is what they found".
These are the people, that had the same feeling, the same problem, the same objection. And this (you show them your treatment solution) is their conclusion.

So: "Dear patient. I understand how you feel, other patients felt the same way. And they found that it was so worth to do this treatment, that they thought they should have done it years before."

This is the three steps way to handle objections. Of course, you don't have to do it like a robot. You have to do it in a natural way. If you train it enough, it comes easily.

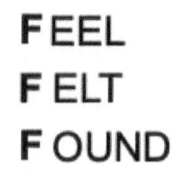

FEEL
FELT
FOUND

19
3 REASONS WHY PATIENTS
BUY YOUR TREATMENTS

In this chapter, I want to talk to you about three reasons why patients buy your treatments.

If you know these three reasons you can cater to them. You promote these three reasons and make people say more "yes" to your treatment offers.

Reason number one.

Patients buy because of emotions, and then they justify it with logic.

They don't buy because of logic, they buy because of emotions. It feels good, it feels right. I buy it! And then they need to justify themselves for this emotional decision.

And they justify it with logic.

You have to paint the picture in their mind. You have to let them feel, they already had that treatment like veneers for example. They should feel like they smile with these beautiful teeth. Paint a picture in the mind first. And then they feel it, they have the emotions of it.

And they will decide based on these emotions, let the conversation feel right. So, if everything flows easily and it's happy and it's going well with the conversation between you and the patient, then this helps the patient to make an emotional decision.

Give them later guidance to see the urgency. Also help them to see what happens, if they do not do the treatment right now. This is also very emotional, but starting to be logic.

And then later, give them also the benefits for a logic justification. Give them all the benefits of the treatment. So that they can justify their emotional decision to make the treatment with you.

Reason number two.

Patients don't buy their way into something, but they buy a way out of something.

Not into something, what does that mean? They do not *want* the treatment. Who wants dental treatment? Nobody wants dental treatment.

They want a way out of their problem. This is what they buy. They do not buy veneers. They buy a way out of their ugly smile.

This is something very important to understand. If you understand that, you focus more on their needs, on their problems on their pain. Not physical, but psychological pain.

They have a problem, you give them the solution. The treatment is the solution to that problem. Let them be aware of their problem. Paint a picture in their mind, not only of the outcome, also of their problem. Are there future problems involved? Are they possible with that problem that they have right now?

That is how you create a little bit of urgency and present the treatment as the solution to their pain. Their pain in the neck, just graphically speaking.

You help them to get out of this pain in the neck.

Reason number three.

Patients don't buy products or services. They buy stories.

Much more than products or services? What does that mean? That means you have to add a story to treatment.

Here are some ideas on how you add a story to a treatment.

How did you get started with that treatment? You can tell them how you did your first implant back in 1994. And since then, the techniques have evolved a lot there is a lot of new technology that has come out in the market and nowadays, we don't use the same technology you used in 1994. You paint a picture in the mind of the patient that you have a story with implantology. Or with smile design, or periodontology, orthodontic treatments, Invisalign™, or whatever.

You just have to tell the patient about your experience with it and then it becomes a story. It now is not only a treatment, but a treatment with a story, *your* story.

Another possibility would be to tell the patient why you do it. Why did you choose to do orthodontic treatments or periodontal treatments? To help patients of course. But you have to tell him then stories of people that you have treated well: "I had this patient and he wrote me a letter a few years later, thanking me for having made his smile design because he got a good job, just because of his smile".

Just a small story about a patient, who was in the same (mental) pain as your patient is now, and now got out of that pain. This story makes the patient decide more towards your treatment than towards the treatment of another dentist.

Tell (real) stories and sell (real) treatments.

20
START CLOSING, DON'T SELL
YOUR TREATMENTS

In this chapter, we will talk about a simple idea on how to start closing and how not to appear you are selling your treatments.

There is a big difference between a salesperson, and a closer and you have to know about it. A simple idea is based on the concept of value in advance.

There is one business truth. You don't get paid by selling. You only get paid when you close a sale. So don't sell, close!

The difference between a salesperson and a closer is this:
If you think about a salesperson, what comes to your mind? In my mind, it's like pushy, sounds aggressive, it's scammy. That's an old concept of a salesperson. The difference between an old-fashioned salesperson and a closer is, when the patient ends up saying "thank you" after he has made the purchase.

Closers help patients to make the correct decision. You have to see yourself as a good closer.

Value in Advance

One simple idea to make the close easier is the formula, which is called Value in Advance. It implies a lot of work before you even talk to the patient, so the patient is already sold on you. On you and your treatment.

Before he comes to you. Then the close is easy for you. That's the idea.

You have to give value in advance, so that he is already sold on anything you might propose to him.

How do you do that in dentistry? What is the best way to sell a box of chocolate? You give them a small piece of chocolate to take. Then they like it, and they buy the whole box of chocolate.

What can you do in advance?

You can make a digital smile design, for example, take a picture of the patient, and you design a digital smile. The patient sees himself with a new smile. That would be value in advance.

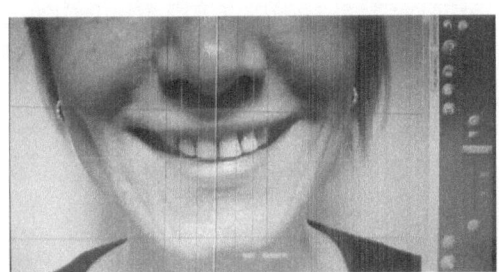

If you don't have a digital smile design software, what you can do is a wax-up. Show them how it could look like. You make an impression, you send it to the lab, and the lab makes a wax-up.

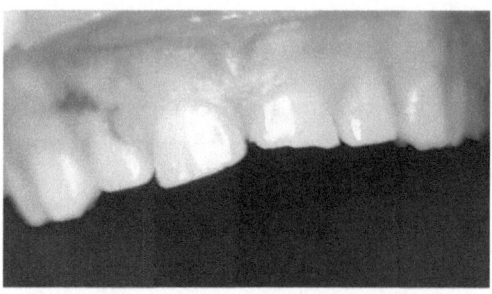

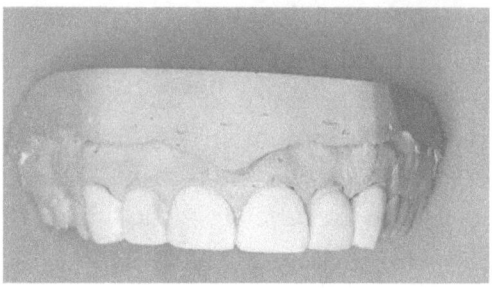

If that isn't enough, you can make an impression (putty) of that wax-up and fill it in with a temporary crown and bridge material and then you put it on the patient's mouth and let it get hard. Like a mock-up, show them in their mouth, how it could look. This picture here is a patient with a mock-up in the mouth.

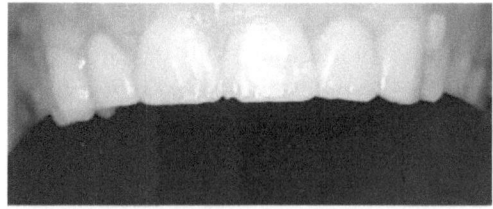

Based on a wax-up all these things are things that you can do in advance.

There is a great idea, that I found in the United States. It's the Smile Virtual Consult™ by Dr. Brian Harris.

He has invented that method. It is simply genius. He has set up a system of value in advance.

The patient sends his pics and his wishes to his email. He makes a video explaining the options and showing before and afters of similar situations he has done.

The patient is immediately convinced. That makes Dr. Harris and the dentists in his system very successful. Patients fly hours across the continent in the United States and Canada to get the treatment done in his office.

This combines your branding with patient education and marketing in one. Now it nearly becomes an automatic closing. The patient, who comes in is already sold on it. Now, you just have to fine-tune the conditions. The closing is natural, not forceful, and patients are happy to be closed.

You can contact Dr. Brian Harris to be one of the doctors in his system and he will help you through all these steps and implement his system in your office.

There is another business truth.

Closing is not something that you do **with** somebody, closing is something that you do **for** somebody.

Keep that in mind and you will be a successful closer.

21
STEPS TO IMPROVE YOUR SALES PROCESS

In this chapter, we will talk about the steps to improve your sales process in your dental clinic.

You will learn the five steps for your sales process.

You will get to know the patient's perspective and how to improve that process.

Your sales process is one side of the medal. It is your perspective. When you think about the sales process, it's how **you** see it.

But there is another way of seeing it. It's the patient's view. The other side is the patient's experience. It's his or her perspective.

Step one.

Prospecting or lead generation to find new patients.

That's your marketing campaign. That's the content marketing, your blogs, whatever you post on social media. Your advertisement.

But from the patient's perspective, it's awareness. They get aware of you. Make them aware that you even exist.

The sales process starts with: they don't know you. And then the first step is to make them aware of you.

Step two.

Qualifying the leads, it's a filtering process.

A lot of people are now aware of you, but not all of them are your ideal patient or need your treatments.

You need to filter them, and you filter them in three ways.

-   The needs. How strong are their needs? Do they really need a smile-makeover? Do they really need now an implant or orthodontic treatment?
-   The time. How urgent is their problem in their mind? Do they want to solve it right now? You can also project that into their mind with your advertisement, with your blogging, with your post on social media. You can make them feel urgent about a certain problem.
-   The money. Are they able to buy the treatment? What resources do they have? Do they have a budget for it? Who has the budget for dentistry? Nobody, so: can they afford what you're selling?

You need to focus your posts, and your blogging and your advertisements to these three things. And then only by your advertisement or only by your blogging or posting on Instagram and Facebook and Twitter, you are already filtering patients. So only the patients that qualify for these three things now continue to stay with you.

From a patient's perspective, that means it's engagement. They are engaging now with your service or your clinic.

So first they are aware, and then now they engage, they want to find out a little bit more about you. They need more information about you to engage more, you need to make sure you offer that information.

They don't know you, you make them aware of you, and now they start to engage with you.

Step three.

Demonstrating value.

You have to walk them through the elaboration process, for example, how to make an implant or other treatments. You make small videos, showing them how you do the implants.

The surgery process (show no blood or cut), the impression taking, the cementation of the final crown or the final restoration. How you do veneers and so on. Make small videos about that or small posts to show how you do the things so that makes them more valuable for the patient.

Show them before and afters, so that they see and think: "this dentist can help me. I have also that same situation. And this is how the other patient got his beautiful smile, so he can help me also".

Testimonials. Present what you can do for the patient. All these things demonstrate value.

From the patient's perspective, it means interest.

Now he or she starts to be interested in your treatment.

Let's go through the process how it goes until now:

At first, they don't know you, then you make them aware of you, then they engage with you and now they are interested in you.

Step four.

Negotiate and close.

They come to your clinic, you present your solution for their case. And now you have to talk about terms of payment, terms of financing, the dates and length of treatment, and so on.

Establish expectations so you don't over-promise. Never over-promise. Just say "this is what we're going to do. And these are the steps and here is how you will look like. You will be restored temporarily for this amount of time". Now the patient knows what to expect.

"You will be a little bit uncomfortable right after the surgery. That's why we give you some medications". All these things, so that the patient knows.
- What's the process?
- How is it going to be?
- How will I have to pay for that?
- What can I expect?

From the patient's view, that is already to get to a commitment (this is what I want and this is how I get it).

Make it very clear for the patient, then the patient engages with you.

So first they don't know you, then you make them aware, they engage with you, they are interested in you, and now they commit.

Step five.

Delivery and fulfillment.

Here is where you get the referrals from and the repeated business of the patient.

It's your service. It's how you deliver your promise. How you deliver your treatment and how you fulfill the completed treatment. How is the end result?

But the sale doesn't stop after you close.

From the patient's perspective, that's the experience.

What is the experience you are providing for your patient? This is what you have to remind yourself in this step.

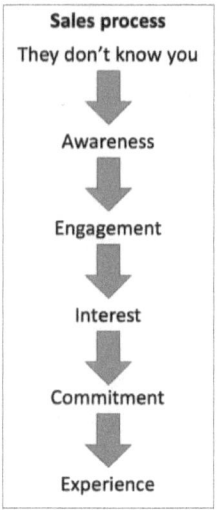

That's the whole sales process.

- They don't know you.
- Then you make them aware with good content. Good content on Instagram, on Facebook, social media, YouTube, blogs, publications, advertisements and so on.
- Then they engage with you. You provide them information about yourself, in social media and in your website.
- Then they become interested in you, you have to build value. Before and afters, testimonials and so on.
- Then they commit with you, you have to set clear expectations. Then the commitment is easy.
- And then you deliver the experience of your patient service. The Ritz Carlton™ experience in your office makes, that they refer to you more and more patients and they come in over and over again, them and their families.

ABOUT THE AUTHOR

Dr. Gómez is Spaniard and **D.D.S., M.D. and Ph.D.** from the University of Tübingen, **Germany**.

For the past 25 years, Dr. Gómez has been in **tight contact with the dental industry**. He worked in the headquarters of a big dental corporation for three years.

In the last 20 years, Dr. Gómez has held **over 400 lectures**, seminars and hands-on workshops in 42 different countries all over the world, **many of them in Dental Business Management**.

After some years in the most prestigious dental offices of Germany,
Dr. Gomez finally moved to Spain in 2004, where he runs his dental office in Valencia, Spain, focusing on **Esthetic Dentistry and Implants**.

Spain is an extremely hostile environment to run a dental office as a business, due to the legislation and the overflow of dental universities. Starting from scratch and succeeding in that environment gives the book a higher value.

www.ingramcontent.com/pod-product-compliance
Lightning Source LLC
Chambersburg PA
CBHW030950240526
45463CB00016B/2325